INTERMITTENT FASTING TO UNLOCK HIDDEN POTENTIALS

The Ultimate Step-by-Step Guide to Slow Down Aging, Undergo Fast and Easy Weight Loss, and Improve your Overall Quality of Life Through the Process of Metabolic Autophagy

Dr. Leonard Cain

© Copyright 2019 - All rights reserved.

The content contained within this book may not be reproduced, duplicated or transmitted without direct written permission from the author or the publisher.

Under no circumstances will any blame or legal responsibility be held against the publisher, or author, for any damages, reparation, or monetary loss due to the information contained within this book, either directly or indirectly.

Legal Notice:

This book is copyright protected. It is only for personal use. You cannot amend, distribute, sell, use, quote or paraphrase any part, or the content within this book, without the consent of the author or publisher.

Disclaimer Notice:

Please note the information contained within this document is for educational and entertainment purposes only. All effort has been executed to present accurate, up to date, reliable, complete information. No warranties of any kind are declared or implied. Readers acknowledge that the author is not engaging in the rendering of legal, financial, medical or professional advice. The content within this book has been derived from various sources. Please consult a licensed professional before attempting any techniques outlined in this book.

By reading this document, the reader agrees that under no circumstances is the author responsible for any losses, direct or indirect, that are incurred as a result of the use of the the information contained within this document, including, but not limited to, errors, omissions, or inaccuracies.

Table of Contents

Description

Have you been trying to slim down unsuccessfully? Have you starved for days and weeks, only to regain all of the weight with crash dieting? If this is true, *"Intermittent Fasting to Unlock Hidden Potentials"* is the right book for you! In this book, you will learn:

- What is Intermittent Fasting;
- How to use it to your advantage;
- Why you're failing to lose weight despite doing the best you can to eat healthily;
- What are the true healing capacities of your own body, and how to eat to unlock the body's hidden potentials;
- How to trigger fast and permanent weight loss;
- How conventional dieting causes insulin resistance, and what you can do to start burning fat instead of your muscles to lose weight;
- How to fast easily and effectively while being full and satisfied;
- How to lose weight without calorie restriction;
- How to eat trigger Autophagy, the powerful process of self-healing, and
- How to recover from cardiometabolic diseases using the right foods.

" *Intermittent Fasting to Unlock Hidden Potentials* " uses a scientific approach to present you with explanations for the most common causes of weight gain and health problems related to diet, such as:

- Obesity as a result of insulin resistance;
- Cardiometabolic disorders as a result of a maladjusted, habitual diet;
- Insulin resistance and its effects on metabolism and weight gain.

Furthermore, " *Intermittent Fasting to Unlock Hidden Potentials* " will give you a thorough explanation of fasting, its origins and history, and the physiological reactions that happen as a result of it. In this book, you will learn about numerous scientifically verified benefits of fasting. You will learn how Intermittent Fasting can help you:

- Lose weight permanently with a simple, sustainable, and satisfying diet plan;
- Cure insulin resistance and turn your body into a fat-burning machine;
- Schedule your meals and exercises to grow muscle mass and burn the fatty tissue;
- Change your diet to support cardiovascular health and improve well-being;

- Identify how your diet affects your health and find the right strategies to support your health with natural foods;
- Learn how to use diet to strengthen your immune system, brainpower, and muscle power; and
- How to enhance the benefits of fasting by going on the Keto diet.

Preface

I wrote this book in hopes of promoting a healthy, safe, and easy diet that will fit everyone. One of the things that intrigued me the most was the potential the fasting has to help the body unlock its self-healing mechanism. With the years of work in the field of nutrition under my belt, I have met many people who felt confused and lost about their diet. The idea of Intermittent Fasting intrigued my mind, and I decided to use a scientific approach to create a guidebook that will help you lose weight, purify the body, and feel well and energized.

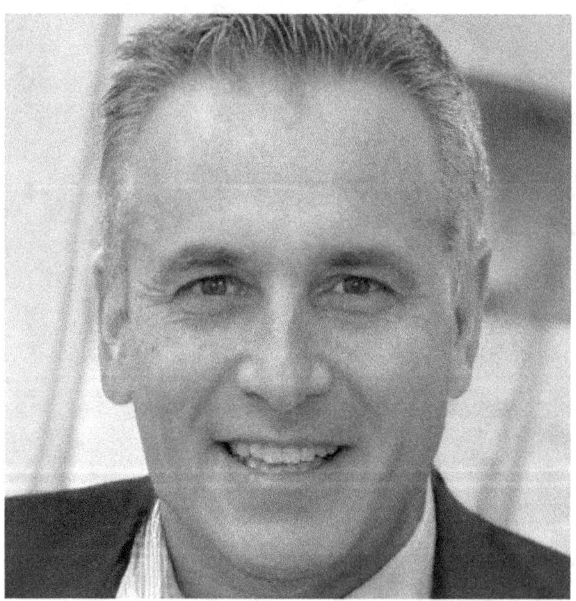

Introduction

The conventional way of eating, which means having three larger meals, and one or multiple snacks each day, hasn't been necessary for a human to survive and stay healthy throughout evolution. The history of fasting has a lot to do with the availability of food, and the spiritual practices of ancient civilizations.

First and foremost, ancient humans didn't have a consistent supply of food throughout the year. It wasn't uncommon for people to eat only one meal per day, and it was also common for days to go by without families having anything to eat. Fasting was present in human history in two main forms:

- Unintentional fasting that resulted from either lacking food or lacking time to eat; and
- Intentional fasting, which was a part of religious, spiritual practices.

What we might call "unintentional fasting," meaning an extended period without consuming food, resulted from periods of devastation, like disease, war, drought or extreme weather. Before modern civilization offered the advantages of cheap and available foods, people also adjusted their diet to seasonal foods. The diet was usually rich and abundant in spring and summer, while the winter months often meant going by on scarce food supplies. These limitations disappeared with the development of farming and agriculture, but the busy lives of the common folk who've spent entire days working often meant that they ate only once or twice per day. Even when the food supplies were no longer brought into question, fasting remained a common practice.

Intentional, or better yet spiritual fasting, was a common practice of ancient cultures and religions. Almost every culture and religion propagates some form of fasting. Spiritually, the fast has the purpose of cleansing and purifying the body. The earliest records of fasting are found in Ancient Greece, where it was used as a purifying and healing tradition.

Nowadays, almost every major religion practice fasting. It is present in Christianity (mainly Orthodox), Buddhism, and Islam. Modern science is now examining and confirming the beliefs that range back thousands of years into human history.

However, the interest in Intermittent Fasting had spread beyond the medical field. The diet is now attracting attention for its convenience, flexibility, weight-loss effectiveness, and healing capacities. In this book, we will review and explain the concept of Intermittent Fasting, while offering practical and useful advice for incorporating the diet into your daily life.

Chapter 1: Explanation of Intermittent Fasting

Fasting as a part of cultural and religious practices involves restricting meals to early morning and evening, which is similar to Intermittent Fasting (the food is consumed during a specified feeding window). In this chapter, you will learn more about Intermittent Fasting, the metabolic processes behind it, and the right ways to follow the regime.

What is Intermittent Fasting?

Intermittent Fasting, as the name suggests, promotes fasting during a limited window of time. When you're fasting, your resting energy expenditure (the amount of calories burned while you're not eating) increases. This means that your body switches from using glucose from your blood to create energy to using fat. When you have access to burning fat supplies, your metabolism works faster because you're not in a calorie deficit.

Glucagon, which is a pancreatic hormone that has a similar effect on insulin, will rise around four to five hours after you've eaten. The nutrients that you've digested have all been stored and used. The purpose of glucagon will now be to supply your body with glucose and feed your brain and red blood cells. It will do it by breaking down the carbohydrates that you've stored inside your body and also by using the leftover fragments of protein from your liver. It will also activate the hormone-sensitive lipase, which will trigger fat to be released from your fat cells and allow other cells in your body to be fueled by fat instead of glucose.

This means that when you fast, your belly fat gets turned into energy that maintains your organs and muscles. This process slows down when you are constantly snacking, which is why reducing the feeding window is recommended.

I came across many studies that showed that time-restricted feeding led to a reduction of body fat and positively impacted impaired fasting glycemia (Hamilton, 2017). When you have impaired fasting glycemia, it means that your blood glucose is higher than normal when you're not eating. This is dangerous because blood sugar should below once you've digested your food. These studies have not only revealed that Intermittent Fasting helps you regulate blood glucose, but they've also detected metabolic and anthropometric improvements, which meant that the study participants:

- Improved their metabolism,
- Showed significant improvements in weight loss and body composition, and
- Improved overall health.

How do You Lose Weight When You're Fasting?

Intermittent Fasting is not about starving your body, but rather having all of your daily food within your daily feeding window so that for the rest of your day, there are no foods ingested. As a result of this, the mechanisms and biological reactions that result from eating are contained to that eating window and not being triggered during the fasting window.

Despite the general knowledge, research shows that having meals less often boosts the metabolic rate. This means that the premise that you need multiple, five to six, or even seven smaller meals during the day to stay slim is wrong. Intermittent Fasting is based on the premise that having spent a certain amount of time every day without eating will trigger the fat burning because no new foods are being introduced into your body.

When you lose weight naturally, it won't slow down your basal metabolic rate. The basal metabolic rate is the number of calories you burn while resting. It greatly depends on your weight, gender, height, and age, and has a lot to do with your lean muscle mass.

Fasting Burns Fat, Not Muscles

Despite the studies showing a significant weight loss during Intermittent Fasting, the question remained whether the weight loss pertains to fat loss or muscle loss. One study that focused on the Ramadan fast detected a 2% muscle loss at the end of the holiday. As a result of an inadequate diet during the feeding times, the participants burned muscle tissue instead of fat. Their weight reduced, but the amount of fat inside their bodies stayed the same.

It was the insufficient protein in the diet, detected in the studies, that had led to the loss of lean body mass. The reduction of fat storage was insignificant. Studies have also revealed many indicators of malnutrition, such as the decrease in albumen protein and overall dehydration. Fasting glucose levels elevated by 11.15%, despite the fact that participants spent nearly 24-hours between meals.

During the month of Ramadan, greater amounts of sweet foods and carbohydrates were consumed compared to protein and fats. Combined with decreased physical activity, it is the reason why weight loss was only temporary. While Intermittent Fasting can cause temporary weight loss regardless of the food you're eating, you can only lose lean muscle mass if you base your diet on carbohydrates. If you don't persist with the diet for longer periods of time, balance out your diet to have sufficient protein and fats, and stay physically active, you will regain your weight.

Fasting Targets Abdominal Fat

There are multiple types of fat cells. Abdominal or visceral fat surrounds your internal organs, while the subcutaneous fat is below the surface of the skin. Having fat supplies in the abdominal area increases your risk of heart disease, diabetes, stroke, high blood pressure, and other illnesses. It has been proven that abdominal fat cells produce more hormones and biochemicals that affect health, such as Cytokines. Cytokines are known to increase the risk of cardiovascular disease because they promote low-level inflammation and insulin resistance.

Different forms of fat have a different effect on the body and require specific dietary efforts to get burned. Subcutaneous and visceral adipose tissue depots are found beneath the skin and can be divided into the upper (stomach) and lower (gluteal and femoral) depots.

Your lean muscle mass burns more energy while you rest. The more muscle you have, the more calories you burn when you are resting, and you lose more muscle when losing weight. When your diet strategy is to avoid proteins, it will slow down your metabolism. When you fast, your body releases growth hormones that encourage your body to use other fuel sources, belly fat among them, instead of muscle mass. When you've triggered the release of growth hormones, your body will resort to burning fat. The growth hormone is also related to the growth hormone IGF1, which is similar to insulin but helps your muscles build more protein.

For you to burn belly fat, there are three types of free fatty acids that need to be released out of your fat cells within a process called lipolysis; then, they need to move into your bloodstream and get transferred into the mitochondria of your cells. After this, they are burned through the process is known as cell oxidation.

How to Follow Intermittent Fasting

Following Intermittent Fasting is simple and convenient. The diet itself doesn't focus on food, but on the timing of the meals. However, for your diet to be successful, you'll need to abide by a couple of general rules:

No Calorie Restriction

Intermittent Fasting has attracted interest for its premise that people don't have to restrict calories every day to lose weight. Studies on humans and animals have used protocols of fasting that included fasting intervals from 20-36 hours. This means that during this time, there was no food ingested. A small amount of food intake with energy restriction of at least 70%, called "modified fasting" (fasting that only takes place two-three days of the week), has been proven effective for weight loss. However, this doesn't mean that you need to cut calories to lose weight. Instead, you can reduce calories on specific days, when it suits your schedule, and eat normally for the remainder of the week.

No Food Restriction

Experts who've studied Intermittent Fasting reported weight loss in overweight, obese, and healthy overweight of 4-10% throughout 4-24 weeks, regardless of the food used in the diet. While the differences in the foods used in the studies often make it difficult to compare the results, the consistent weight loss detected despite all of the differences suggests that the choice of foods doesn't have a dramatic impact on the diet results.

No Lifestyle Adjustments

While there's still a large debate on the best approach to weight loss, a steady, moderate, sustainable diet with abidance to the plan has been proven to yield the best results. While the research data doesn't support that Intermittent Fasting is easy, it shows it's acceptable, sustainable, and most importantly, effective.

How Intermittent Fasting Works

The human body can be either in a "fasting" or "fed" state. These are the main two stages of your metabolism that align with the two main metabolic processes:

- Catabolism, and
- Anabolism.

During catabolism, you are breaking down the foods you're consuming. This process breaks down the food molecules into smaller particles that release energy. Once the food particles have been broken down to supply energy, the anabolic process begins. Now, your body will use the energy to maintain tissues, organs and body functions, and to repair the cells of your body. While these processes happen simultaneously, they can happen at different rates. The conventional way of eating stimulates catabolism vs anabolism, slowing down the rate in which your body nourishes and repairs itself. When you're fasting, your body has more time for the second stage of metabolism.

Fasting gives you a metabolic advantage because the body burns fat as long as it doesn't detect calorie deficit. Avoiding calorie restriction will be greatly highlighted throughout this book since calorie restriction has been proven to slow down metabolism even in otherwise healthy people.

To lose weight, you need to spend more calories than you consume. Negative energy balance happens when a person spends a greater amount of calories than they consume. This is a no-brainer. However, this fact has also caused people to believe that the best way to lose weight is to eat as less as possible. This inaccurate assumption was debunked by many studies that didn't show any differences in body weight before and after the calorie restriction.

Intermittent Fasting Stimulates the Release of Ketones

Ketone bodies serve as a source of energy during fast. Ketones are produced in the liver from fatty acids, which are mobilized and distributed through blood circulation to active tissues, like the brain and muscles. Ketones can regulate cellular functions, which affects cardiometabolic disease risks. They can contribute to improving cardiometabolic health by:

- Improving the function of skeletal muscle and mitochondria,(cellular parts that break down old components and turn them into energy) and
- Regulating insulin sensitivity.

What is the main benefit of Intermittent Fasting?

The most important benefit of Intermittent Fasting can be summed up in one sentence:

When you are fasting, your body burns fat more than it usually does.

Fasting allows your body to release energy for you to use throughout the day, but it does that by burning your fat storage. As a result of this, you are:

- Losing weight;
- Getting rid of excess fat from your body; and
- Triggering the healing processes inside your body (autophagy and hormesis) that will be discussed in the later chapters.

When the time between meals is prolonged, your body has more time to return to balance and start burning fat. This improves your natural sensitivity to insulin. Fasting also reduces inflammation, which happens as a response of your body to injuries. Inflammation has a purpose to remove the cause of the injury and to start the healing process. However, too much inflammation is dangerous in conditions such as eczema and arthritis. When you have high levels of body fat, your inflammatory markers will also increase.

Intermittent Fasting allows you to follow a consistent diet regimen without having to follow a specific eating pattern. It is simple to plan and execute, and not very demanding in regard to meal planning and food preparation. You will simply limit the daily food intake to a feeding window and divide that time across different meals, which is easier to follow than specific times and structures of the meal. Studies have shown that obese patients benefit from feeling full and satisfied, which helped them stop overeating on non-fasting days.

Chapter 2: Autophagy

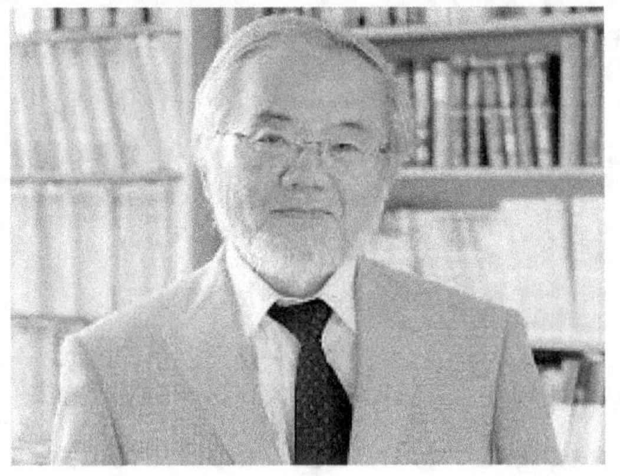

Autophagy is a naturally-occurring process in your body that triggers in a fasted state. It happens when your body breaks down its own old cells to create energy and uses that energy to grow new, healthy cells. It is a process during which your body gets rid of old, unhealthy tissues. When you are in a state of fast, your body doesn't only use fat to supply energy. It also starts using the old, defective cells. In 2016, Yoshinori Ohsumi, a Japanese scientist, won the Nobel Prize in Physiology or Medicine for his discovery of autophagic mechanisms. Scientists worldwide are now using his discoveries to study how autophagy can help cure diseases and promote health.

What is Autophagy?

Autophagy is an ancient mechanism or pathway of self-digestion through lysosomal degradation. Lysosomal degradation is a process through which the lysosomes, one of the key components of the cells, break down dead parts of cells. Through this process, old and dysfunctional parts of cells are being recycled. One of the more significant Ohsumi's findings states that this process can be both non-selective and selective. Non-selective autophagy happens during nutrient deprivation, when the body breaks down its muscle tissue to supply energy, while selective autophagy happens when the body breaks down damaged parts of cells, such as pathogens and organelles (Levine & Klionsky, 2017).

The term roughly "autophagy" roughly translates to "self-eating." As the name suggests, your body "eats" (breaks down into energy) its own cells and tissues to heal itself. During the process of autophagy, your body gets rid of all unnecessary cells and tissues, including excess skin. Those who've lost significant amounts of weight with autophagy and Intermittent Fasting reportedly didn't have issues with excess skin.

Autophagy and Mitochondrial Dysfunction

You can think of autophagy as a process in which your body replaces all defective mitochondria (cellular parts that are in charge of the energy output) that are now losing its function, with the healthy mitochondria.

Mitochondrial dysfunction links to many diseases, like diabetes and neurological problems. The process of self-eating helps your cells get rid of the damaged mitochondria and allows them to grow and replace them with new mitochondria that are more energy-efficient. It also helps your body heal from all sorts of injuries and fight infections. When you fast, your body eliminates the cells that are dying and those that are already dead. Then, the process of building new cells is being accelerated and stimulated.

When you're in the state of autophagy, you're also getting rid of the toxic waste that is getting in the way of the nourishment of your body. This, in return, helps you normalize your metabolic rate and restore cell oxygenation. Fasting also helps to stabilize your insulin response, reduce inflammation, improve cardiovascular health, and even support cancer treatment.

Autophagy and Aging

To understand how autophagy slows aging, it is important to understand the role of the insulin-like growth factor 1 (IGF 1). IGF-1 is a hormone that works on a cellular level, and it has both positive and negative effects. It is anabolic, which means that it helps your cells grow and multiply. When this hormone is high, your cells will constantly divide and multiply. In order to slow aging and prevent the DNA damage to your cells that can occur due to the long-term influence of an inadequate diet, you want to lower your levels of IGF 1 (Hamilton, 2017).

When your IGF 1 drops, your body will produce new cells in a slower pace and start repairing your old cells. However, when your IGF 1 is too low for longer periods of time, it will cause DNA damage to your cells. This damage is more likely to remain permanent unless you make the right changes to your diet.

Isolation
membrane
Autophagosome
Lysosome
Lysosomal hydrolase
Autolysosome
VESICLE
NUCLEATION
VESICLE
ELONGATION
DOCKING
& FUSION
VESICLE BREAKDOWN
& DEGRADATION

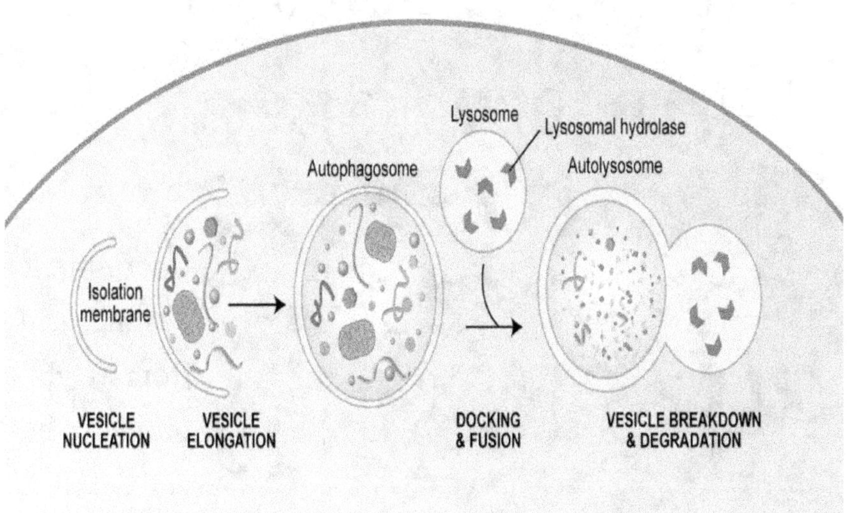

Chapter 3: Benefits of Intermittent Fasting

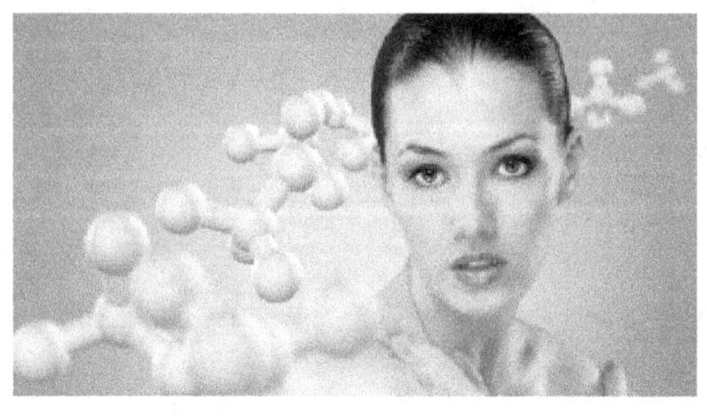

Intermittent Fasting, aside from weight loss, promotes health and delays aging. It increases cognitive functioning and is said to protect against inflammation, neurological diseases, and cancer(Stephens, 2017).

Fasting and Insulin Resistance

Eating a high amount of fat and sugary foods increase your risk of insulin resistance. Insulin resistance increases the risk of diabetes, cancer, cardiovascular disease, and other inflammatory diseases. What science has so far confirmed is that fasting helps control blood sugar. Partial calorie restriction has been proven to raise ketone levels after two days of a 12-hour overnight fast. Simultaneously, the decrease of insulin has been found.

Insulin has a role in both weight loss and weight gain. Insulin controls whether or not your fat supplies will remain stored inside your body, or they'll be used for their intended purpose. Insulin levels are normally low when you're not eating. When your insulin is low, your body starts to burn fat. Low insulin allows you to burn fat for energy. With type 1 diabetes, the insulin-producing cells in the body aren't functioning. Fat stores are burnt to the extreme, and people are unable to gain weight regardless of their food intake. Type 1 diabetes can be fatal if untreated. For these patients, elevating the insulin levels is beneficial because it allows the body to store fat.

Insulin resistance is the opposite of this. Having insulin resistance means that your body produces more insulin than needed. This happens because your cells become less sensitive to insulin, and normal amounts of it can no longer move into the cells. As a result of this, the glucose remains in your blood. To force the glucose into your cells, the body then creates excess amounts of it. The constantly elevated glucose levels then stop fat burning.

The cause of insulin resistance is a vicious cycle of elevated glucose. When the glucose levels elevate, the cells create resistance to protect against the overwhelming influence. Then, greater amounts of insulin are required to fuel cells. The body starts creating more insulin, but the resistance of the cells only increases. The only way to break this vicious cycle is to drastically reduce insulin levels.

The problem with dieting is that the elevated insulin levels combined with calorie restriction only slow down the metabolism. If you don't consume sufficient calories to maintain normal levels of glycogen and your insulin levels are elevated, there's no release of fat cells. When your body can't access the fat storages, nor use the energy from the foods you consume, your metabolism will slow down. This is a way for your body to preserve energy. Fasting is a solution to this. Eating raises insulin, but your body now burns glucose that is available from foods. However, it is important to reduce carbohydrates because they tend to rise insulin the most. The more severe your insulin resistance is, the more you'll need fasting and carbohydrate reduction to jumpstart the metabolism.

When you're fasting, your metabolism stabilizes and your hormones (adrenaline and growth hormones) return to balance. Insulin and blood sugar levels go down as a result.

Studies confirmed these claims, showing that the study groups that had the same calorie intake, but one fasted and the other didn't show differences in insulin and blood glucose levels. The study group that fasted had lower levels of insulin, and improved insulin resistance compared to the group that was on a calorie reduction diet.

Intermittent Fasting Stimulates the Release of Ketones

Ketone bodies serve as a source of energy during fast. Ketones are produced in the liver from fatty acids. Fatty acids are mobilized and distributed through blood circulation to active tissues, like the brain and muscles. Ketones can regulate cellular functions, which affects cardiometabolic disease risks. They can contribute to improving cardiometabolic health by improving the function of skeletal muscle and mitochondria, and regulating the insulin sensitivity.

Fasting Increases Fat Burning

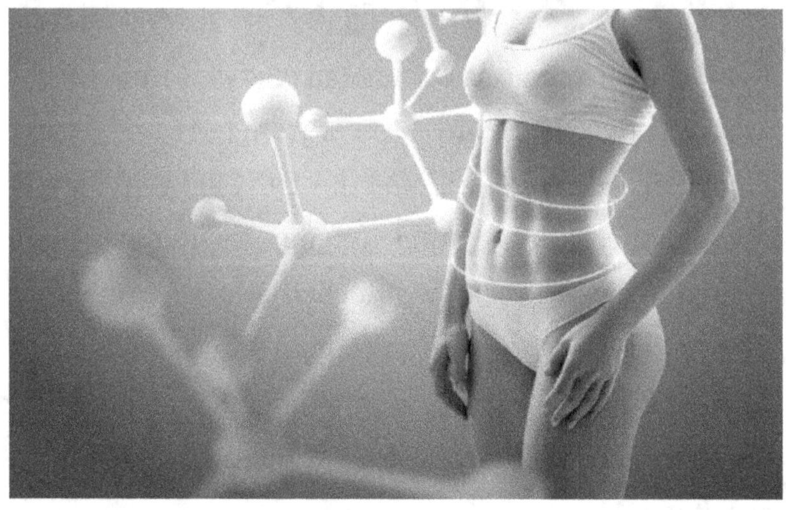

When you fast, the calories you burn to fuel your body and brain come from your fat stores instead of your lean mass and the blood glucose. Because of the release of insulin and glucose into your blood, eating multiple meals across the day will be an effective way of fasting. It will also be useful to preserve your lean muscle. Short-term metabolic adaptation to starvation within 96 hours has been recorded, which shows that the diet becomes effective very fast.

During this process, the glucose is compensated for through the mobilization of liver glycogen stores and the process of gluconeogenesis. The shift in the use of energy, where fat and ketones are used for fuel instead of glucose, which means that your body will start to burn fat rapidly.

Fasting Triggers Hormesis

There's another benefit of fasting that isn't strictly related to diet. It is called "Hormesis." Hormesis is the benefit of putting the body under a small amount of stress. In this case, fasting is the stress that restricts energy to the body. Putting a body under a small, tolerable amount of strain results in an increase of the muscle tissues. This mechanism is similar to the benefits we reap from exercise. When the body goes through a tolerable amount of physical stress, it strengthens its tissues to adjust. Hormesis has been proven to influence the survival of cells and make cells more resistant to heat and oxidative stress.

Hormone and Nutrient Balance

Fasting causes changes in hormones by reducing glucose serum and glycogen that are being stored in the liver. As a result, your body uses ketones and free fatty acids to fuel the brain and body instead of using glucose. This is important for weight loss because when the energy your body uses daily comes from the glucose in your blood, none of the fat supplies are being used. This change has been shown to affect resistance to disease and stress response, resulting in:

- Improved insulin sensitivity,
- Reduction of insulin levels, and

- Improvements in antioxidants and reduction oxidative stress.

The example of "The Daniel Fast" is a good representation of the effect the fasting has on the body. In this fast, foods that are restricted include animal products, processed foods, caffeine, alcohol, sweeteners, and flavors. Instead of fat-dense and processed foods, this diet includes fruits, whole grains, vegetables, seeds, nuts, and oils. The study of this fast showed that those who followed the diet lost around 2.8kg over 21 days without calorie restriction. There was a significant decrease in fat, protein, and an increase in carbohydrates and Vitamin C. There were also improvements in the body composition and metabolism rates, as well as beneficial effects for those who have asthma and cardiovascular disease.

Reduction of free fat mass in women, reduction of total and LDL cholesterol, and reduction in triglyceride levels have also been found in the study participants who've followed this fast. However, there are differences in levels that vary between significant and insignificant when it comes to insulin resistance and insulin sensitivity.

Fasting and Brain Power

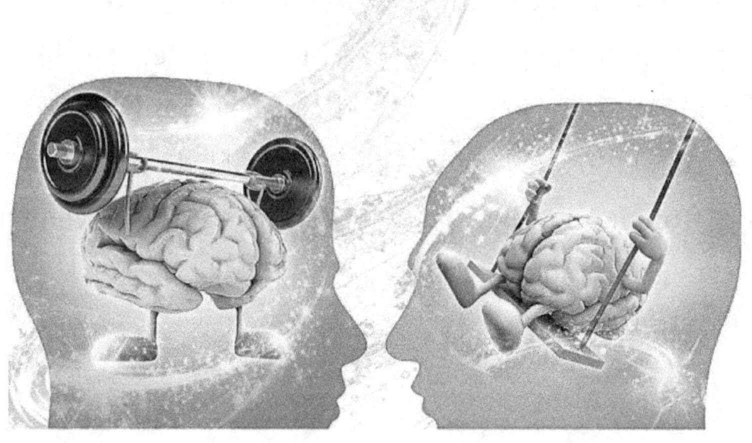

Calorie restriction is proven to impact brain functioning negatively. Studies have shown that fasting won't have a negative impact on brain activity. This is because your body draws the energy from the fat storages, but "knows" that the required amounts of food will come soon, and there's no reason to slow down metabolism. Reduced insulin levels have been found to have beneficial effects on memory and mental abilities, like focusing, attention, reasoning, and abstract thinking.

While there is no evidence that will suggest that fasting will improve your brain health, the food choices might have a lot to do with regaining clarity and a healthy mind. The diet that is rich in vegetables, fruit, fish, olives, and avocados is also associated with good brain health and building muscle mass.

Another benefit of fasting is that it will help mental clarity and make you more aware and better focused. While you're fasting, your body also grows and develops nerve tissues. The more you space out your feeding time, the better the ability of your body to heal and repair itself. On the other hand, the process of autophagy, when triggered, will help transform the energy from fat into the energy that is necessary for your nerves to grow and develop.

Fasting and Heart Health

High blood cholesterol is considered to be a significant risk factor for heart disease. However, not all cholesterol is the same. Cholesterol is responsible for repairing cells and producing vital hormones. What we call "bad" cholesterol is the low-density lipoprotein (LDL), which increases the risk of heart disease, but the "good" cholesterol, high-density lipoprotein (HDL) has beneficial effects on the body without the adverse health effects. The "bad" cholesterol also forms from triglycerides, that are created in the liver due to increased carbohydrate intake. Elevated triglycerides also associated with cardiovascular disease and are also heavily impacted by the diet.

What most people understand wrong is that food intake is responsible for high cholesterol. Studies continue to prove that dietary fat doesn't produce cholesterol. Fasting lowers cholesterol because of the liver synthesizes fewer triglycerides with the reduction of carbohydrates in the diet. Studies have shown that alternate-day fasting through the course of 70 days led to a 25-30% reduction in LDL levels. Why? Because fasting stabilizes the functioning of your liver and balances out the production of triglycerides.

A moderate 5% weight loss found in studies had a significant impact on comorbidities related to obesity. Weight loss improves sensitivity to insulin, blood pressure, glycemic control, and other factors that contribute to the reduction of cardiometabolic risks. Fasting improves your cardiovascular health and circulation by reducing the levels of triglycerides and improving the levels of good cholesterol, such as high-density lipoprotein. High-density lipoprotein helps transport protein that removes excess cholesterol from your bloodstream. Fasting also gives your body and internal setting to increase your resistance to illnesses that are related to age.

Intermittent Fasting and Cancer

Obesity and the symptoms of metabolic syndrome are accounted for being risk factors for cancer. Obesity has been proven to increase the risk of colorectal cancer and to the worsening of the condition in those who are suffering from cancer, including prostate cancer. For those who are suffering from cancer, obesity increases the risk of tumor progression. Also, the increased risks from diabetes and hyperglycemia increase the risk of a fatal outcome for women who are suffering from cancer.

Healthy calorie restriction, combined with a balanced intake of macronutrients, essential fatty acids, and proteins, was found to protect the cells from being exposed to high levels of glucose and other factors that contribute to the growth of cancer cells. As a result, healthy calorie restriction reduces the chance of growing tumors. These studies were mainly done on animals, and there's little proof that the same will happen to humans. However, the studies that have focused on the Japanese people and their eating habits (40% less calorie intake than the average US) have recorded lower cancer rates and average longer life.

Intermittent Fasting has been proven to fight the growth and spread of cancer cells in animals. However, there are no significant studies in humans. What you can be certain is that fasting will activate the mechanisms in your body that are helping it get rid of defective cells and stimulate it to grow new, healthy cells. Studies on animals have also shown that fasting can help improve survival rates after chemotherapy. Research has shown that fasting between one and two days every week might help protect your brain from Parkinson's, Alzheimer's, and other brain diseases. Studies have also shown that food reduction in the short term won't impair your cognitive functions. However, long term calorie restriction will.

Chapter 4: Getting to Know the Facts

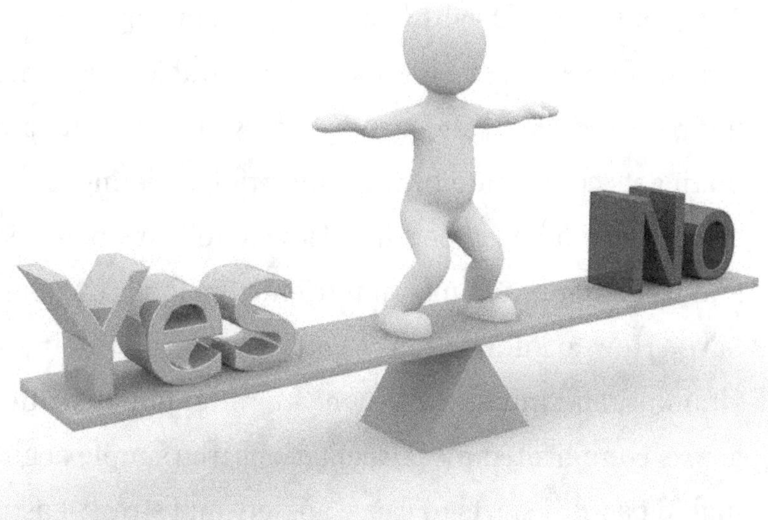

Despite numerous research findings and nearly a century-long use of fasting for medical purposes, there are multiple misconceptions and doubts surrounding Intermittent Fasting. In this chapter, we will review some of the most common misconceptions about fasting, and point out typical errors in dieting. In addition, we will reflect on some of the possible side-effects (Hamilton, 2017).

Myths and Delusions of Intermittent Fasting

Fasting is Difficult

The postulates of healthy eating are seemingly straightforward: eat a lot of fruits, vegetables, lean meat, unprocessed dairy, and avoid processed foods. But simple math gets complicated with conventional dieting. How many calories do you need per day? How to tell how many calories and what amount of macronutrients the foods on your plate have? How to know if you're getting enough protein, vitamins, and minerals? When your attention is scattered across complicated meal calculations, the simple act of making a meal starts to cause anxiety and stress. Fasting makes it simple to understand what kind of diet you need to get better.

With fasting, you are only required to choose a regime that works best for you and focus on eating healthy, clean foods in the amounts you like. Gradually, you can enrich your nutritional knowledge on calories and macronutrients, and start to focus more on the composition of your meals. But, you won't miss out on health benefits if you don't do that. Simply fasting and eating clean will bring significant improvements to your health, and improving your nutritional knowledge will only enhance the benefits.

Fasting is Complicated

Intermittent Fasting doesn't require following a particular meal plan, which makes grocery shopping and meal preparation simple and convenient. Even if you don't have the time to cook at home, eating out won't be a problem for your diet and health. As long as you stay away from fast food, you're good.

Fasting is Restrictive and Isolating

Fasting doesn't require giving up on your favorite treats. Some common-sense limitations apply to those who are recovering from cardiometabolic diseases, but not beyond your doctor's recommendations. Unless you're advised against certain foods, there's no reason to avoid them. Fasting can also be adjusted for you to enjoy social gatherings without having to avoid delicious treats and cocktails. You can always move your feeding window to align with your social activities and go back to your old schedule when convenient.

Easy Weight Loss Sounds Too Good to be True!

Even if you don't trust this book, running a simple search on scientific research on fasting will show you how effective it is. Studies have shown that fasting is beneficial in any form, regardless of whether you choose to apply calorie adjustment and food selection.

Fasting Limits Your Activities

With fasting, you don't have to think about eating the right foods at the right time. This means that you can fast while traveling, at work, or pretty much in any setting. The only thing you need to do is choose the times you'll fast and the times you'll eat, and stick to that decision. Other than that, there are no limitations regarding food choice and meal times.

Additionally, you can fast regardless of your diet preferences. You can fast on a vegan, vegetarian, paleo, ketogenic, and any other diet. Fasting is also effective regardless of whether or not you exercise. The research has shown that fasting won't compromise your capacity to work out, as long as you level the calorie intake with exercise.

How to avoid the common mistakes with Intermittent Fasting

While most people who practice Intermittent Fasting accurately lose weight, many fail. This happens because of diet mismanagement. Here are a couple of ways for you to avoid choosing the wrong type of fast and the wrong foods:

Manage Your Diet Thoughtfully

There are numerous studies on Intermittent Fasting that show promising results, with some pointing out possible negative health consequences after the participants left the study. This highlights the importance of right diet management. The recorded weight loss in study participants was between 2 and 5%, indicating that proper guidance and diet management can make a noticeable difference in weight loss.

Avoid High-Fat Diets

Intermittent low-carb, high-fat, and high-protein fasting diet had similar results as regular Intermittent Fasting. Regardless of weight loss, a high-fat diet can reduce the benefits of the diet and contribute to cardiovascular disease. On the other hand, time-restricted feeding that was based on protein proved beneficial to the overall metabolic health, with improvement of numerous health improvements in metabolism and blood glucose.

Avoid Calorie Restriction

Severe calorie restriction can cause the impairment of glucose tolerance in healthy people. Short and medium Intermittent Fasting didn't worsen glucose tolerance and had led to a 5% weight loss. However, it's a misconception that Intermittent Fasting is more tolerable than regular dieting. Many of the study participants had trouble maintaining a simple, 1000-1500 calorie regimen after the study was over. In addition, Intermittent Fasting didn't seem to cause overeating during feeding times and had also led to a reduction in resting energy expenditure, which is the number of calories burned while the participants were inactive.

Monitor your health

Health benefits of Intermittent Fasting accumulate over time, but there's an increased risk of complications for those who are treating from type 2 diabetes. People who are treating type 2 diabetes are at risk of hypoglycemia. To prevent hypoglycemia when fasting, it is important to monitor blood tests, blood pressure, and vital signs.

Side Effects of Intermittent Fasting

The Risks From Extreme Fasting

Long term fasting can help weight loss and be beneficial for high blood pressure, and it can also help chemotherapy patients. However, there are some dangers and risks from long term fasting that occur if the diet is taken to the extreme. There are numerous health risks involved with prolonged fasting. Fasting for longer than 72 hours can be life-threatening due to nutrient deprivation and dehydration.

Severe Calorie Deprivation

Calorie deprivation is one of the possible risks of Intermittent Fasting. Fasting for a long time stresses your heart as it puts a strain on the cardiac muscle to get fuel. While your body will switch to using fat, the utilization of muscle mass will continue even while the fat reserves are available. This also includes the muscle of your heart. For this reason, I recommend fasting only under the guidance of medical experts, especially if you choose longer periods of fasting per day (e.g., more than 18 hours).

Heart Failure

Extreme fasting can lead to heart failure. This also includes strict water fasting. Strict water fasting can deplete your body of magnesium and potassium, which can also lead to the weakening of your heart muscle, resulting in heart failure.

The weakening of the Immune System

It is also possible to catch numerous infectious diseases due to inadequate nutrition. If your immune system weakens, you can get all sorts of infections. Fasting has a detoxifying effect, and toxins, when removed from the body, can cause uncomfortable symptoms. You could feel nauseous, fatigued, and sick.

Refeeding Syndrome

The refeeding syndrome can happen approximately 1-2 days after an extended fast, when the body may start to break down protein to supply energy. The refeeding syndrome occurs when phosphorus and other electrolytes are depleted. When refeeding begins, the foods you eat will raise insulin, which will then stimulate the synthesis of protein, glycogen, and fat. This will require phosphorus and other minerals, which can result in weakness, fatigue, cramps, tremors, or even seizures. However, it is very rare (less than 0.43% chance) and unlikely to occur in those with sufficient fat supplies to ensure energy.

Chapter 5: Intermittent Fasting Methods

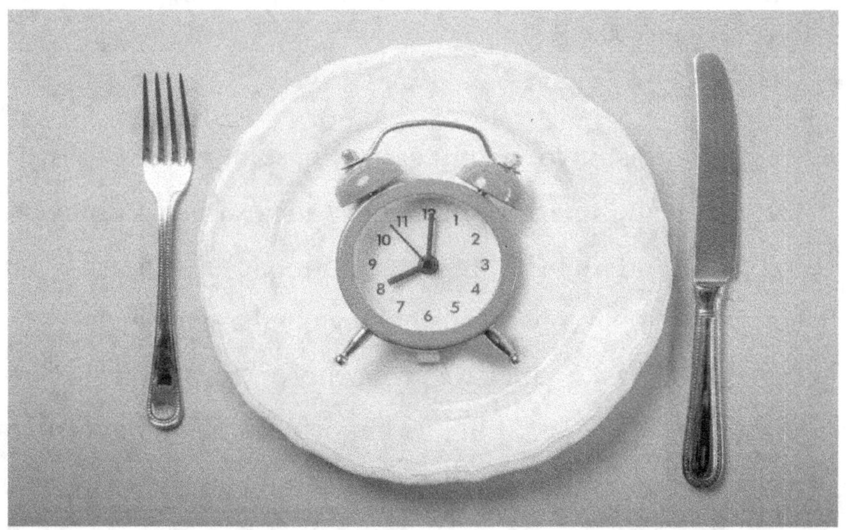

Choosing the right Intermittent Fasting method is the first step toward successful fasting. In this chapter, we will review numerous types of fasting, leaving it up to you to decide which is the most convenient. You can't make a wrong choice, as all of the methods have a proven track record of success (Moore & Fung, 2017).

The 12-Hour Fasting

The 12-hour fast is what you would call a conventional eating pattern, where you fast for 12 hours, and spread your meals across the remaining 12. The advantage of the 12-hour fast is that it introduces a period of very low insulin throughout the day, which prevents insulin resistance. While the 12-hour fast is a good solution for those looking to prevent cardiometabolic disorders, it is not efficient enough to reverse the existing health disorders.

The 24-Hour Fasting

A 24-hour fast involves not eating for 24 hours straight. The fast starts at dinnertime and ends the next day at dinnertime. Keep in mind that fasting for 24 hours doesn't mean starvation. It simply means having one large meal every 24 hours. This fast is convenient for those who are busy throughout the day. Still, it is important to be thoughtful of nutritive values that are being consumed during a single daily meal. It is still important that there's variety in foods, and sufficient calories to avoid starvation.

When fasting for longer times, it is important not to calorie restrict during feeding times. This way, you will avoid starvation and slowing down of the metabolism. The diet should still be low-carb, high-fat, and unprocessed.

The Leangains Method 16/8

The Leangains method of Intermittent Fasting consists of two phases. There's the 16 hours of fasting time and an eight-hour feeding window. The eight-hour feeding window usually includes three meals. The composition of your meals varies depending on your daily schedule and preferences.

This method is more appropriate for fitness enthusiasts and everyone who works out regularly and intensely. It is recommended to break the fast by eating meat on workout days. You should also have more vegetables and fruit than carbs and fats. When you are exercising, you should prioritize carbs while prioritizing fats is recommended on the days when you are not working out. On all days, you should keep your diet protein-rich. However, the composition and size of your meals will depend on weight goals, age, gender, body fat percentage, and the levels of activity.

Before working out, it's recommended to keep your energy levels high. Meals should be medium-sized. On the days that you're not working out, you should eat fewer calories than you consume on your workout days. However, make sure to reduce the intake of carbohydrates, increasing fibrous vegetables, lean meats, and fruits.

When using this method, you should make the first meal largest and then reduce the size of the meal as the day goes by. Your first meal should contain at least 40% of the total calorie intake for the day. It should also be rich in macronutrients. Make sure to have up to 100 grams of protein, and you can also have fattier meats and fish. However, make sure to make healthy choices and go for salmon and ground beef. The last meal should be a protein source that digests slowly. You can have cottage cheese or eggs. It is also all right to have meat or fish as long as you have enough vegetables to supplement the fiber. Having a well-planned dinner will help you stay full during the fast.

Eat-Stop-Eat

The Eat-Stop-Eat Intermittent Fasting method contains a 24-hour long fast for two days of the week and eating as usual for the other five days of the week. However, it is important to make food choices and meal sizes reasonable. It is still important to stick to your regular schedule during the remainder of the week. This method is good for those who have a busy schedule and find it hard to hold on to a daily routine. With this approach, you can avoid eating on days when you are less active and have greater amounts of food on today's you are active.

The Warrior Diet

The warrior diet method includes fasting for 20 hours and then eating for four hours every day. This diet is inspired by the diet of the warriors, as the name suggests. They would eat little, or wouldn't eat anything at all during the day, and then eat during the night. When practicing the warrior diet, you should have small amounts of dairy, eggs, and raw fruits and vegetables during the day, including non-calorie beverages. After 20 hours, you can have as much food as you want to during the overeating window. However, it is important to have healthy and organic, non-processed foods. The warrior diet hasn't been scientifically researched.

The 36-Hour (Alternate-Day) Fasting

The 36-hour fasting is also known as alternate-day fasting. It has been proven to reduce body mass index and improve the torso-fat composition. With this diet, you will fast for 36 hours and then eat anything you want for 12 hours. Studies have shown that this diet had similar effects as calorie restriction. However, it is still important to eat healthy foods on the feeding day. Alternate-day fasting is also an easy way to maintain the diet and has been proven to be more sustainable. Studies have shown that it did lead to a reduction in the overall intake of calories and was easily tolerated. It had beneficial effects on the cardiovascular system and has shown beneficial changes to body composition throughout six months and longer.

The 48-Hour Fasting

The 48-hour fast involves fasting for 48 hours, for two straight days, and then starting to eat on the third day at dinnertime. During the fast, you can have noncaloric fluids like coffee, black water, tea, and other beverages. It is very important to stay hydrated during this fast. After the fast, food should gradually introduce foods to avoid overstimulating your stomach, which could lead to diarrhea, nausea and bloating. The first meal you take after fast should be a light snack, such as a mouth handful of nuts. After two hours, you can have a small meal.

You should maintain your usual eating schedule during the non-fasting days. However, you should still avoid overeating or eating unhealthy foods. It is recommended to do the 48-hour fast once or twice per month instead of weekly to reap greater health benefits.

The 5:2 Fast

During the 5:2 diets, you will normally eat for five days of the week and restrict your calories to 600 for two days of the week. There are no requirements regarding which foods you should eat, but you should stick to healthy food choices.

Women should have 500 calories, and men should have 600 calories on fasting days. Commonly, fasting is done on Mondays and Thursdays, with 1-3 smaller meals eating normally the rest of the week.

However, one shouldn't eat just any food for the rest of the week. The food intake should be kept within reason.

The 4:3 Fast

The 4:3 Intermittent Fasting plan involves having one day eating whatever you want and then fasting the next, and every other day. The fasting days include one 400-calorie meal and one 100-calorie snack. During the fasting days, you should have a lot of water, coffee, and tea and make sure you have prepackaged healthy meals if you think you will be too busy to cook. The benefits of this diet are that it helps you identify how it feels to be truly hungry. It's also noted that 4:3 fasting helps reduce stomach size. Sticking to protein-rich foods will be beneficial for your health, and eating high-fat food will help balance your sugar levels. You should avoid sweeteners on the opposite side. The diet doesn't give any instructions on how a meal should be planned and structured during the fasting day. This can cause you to make mistakes and use the wrong foods on that day.

Forever Fat Loss

Forever fat loss is an approach that includes having the right foods to lose weight without feeling deprived. This approach advises eating all-natural foods to satisfy cravings and break the addiction to junk food. It is important to eliminate the hidden triggers such as watching TV and staying up late at night. Forever fat loss is practiced by addressing behaviors that are triggering the bad eating habits. It is advised to have the following foods: eggs, turkey, chicken, grass-fed beef, lamb, Alaskan salmon, organic feta cheese, wild shrimp, organic yogurt, coconut cream, bok choy, spinach, whey protein, portobello mushrooms, broccoli, tomatoes, cucumbers, peppers, carrots, onions, avocado, potato berries, extra virgin olive oil, raw cocoa and cinnamon.

Chapter 6: How to Start?

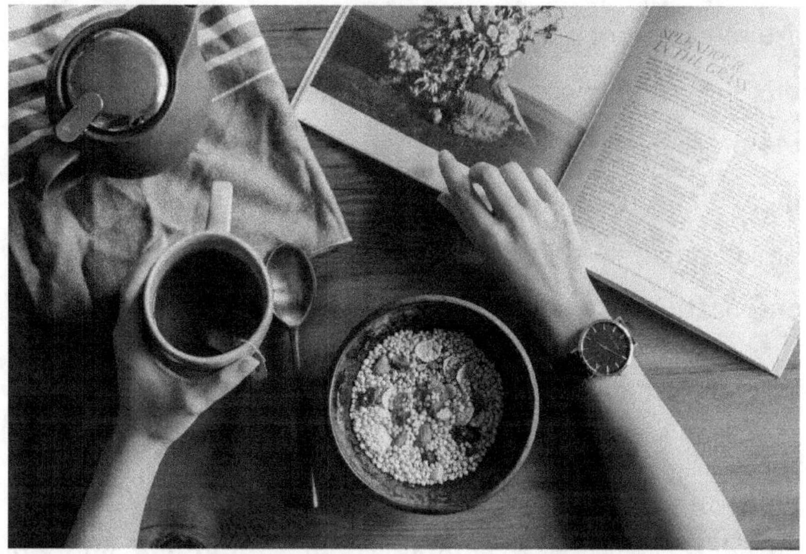

By now, you understand what Intermittent Fasting is, how it works, and the benefits. But, how to start with this diet? In this chapter, I will suggest some tips for you to start fasting and set yourself up for success.

How to Get Started

While Intermittent Fasting isn't difficult, starting a new diet is always a big change. When to start? What to eat? How to eat? In this section, you'll learn what you need to do before you start dieting (Moore & Fung, 2017).

Track Eating Behaviors

The reason that most diets fail is that most of them calculate a desired daily calorie deficit that is based on your initial weight. As you get slimmer, you require a smaller calorie deficit to lose weight. If you stick to the initial number, you are putting more strain on your body than it needs, so your metabolism slows down. Traditional diets are usually hard to maintain because you have to think about mealtimes and meal planning to the degree that makes the diet unsustainable. Also, most diets don't address eating habits and particularly habitual and emotional eating.

Your weight gain could have a lot to do with your eating behaviors. Eating beside any other reason than being physically hungry is wrong. You could be eating out of boredom, stress, or to compensate for unfulfilled emotional needs. The best way for you to determine the reasons why you are overeating is to track your meals, the reasons you thought you were hungry, and what you ate at that time. This approach will help you identify when, how much, and which foods you eat for the wrong reasons. It will make it easier for you to identify the foods you need when you are truly, physically hungry.

Set Goals

A healthy weight loss goal is to lose between one and two pounds every week. If you start losing more, there's a chance that you are losing muscle mass. There's credible research to confirm that it's possible to lose lean muscle mass with Intermittent Fasting if you don't eat enough protein. You can be healthy when it comes to weight but still have high amounts of abdominal fat, which can cause many health risks. The goals with Intermittent Fasting depend on your health and weight goals. You can determine your diet goals by answering a couple of simple questions:

- Which improvements are you seeking? Do you want to:
    - ☐ Reduce the symptoms of illness,
    - ☐ Feel better,
    - ☐ Become more energized,
    - ☐ Lose weight, or
    - ☐ All of the above?
- Are you interested in practicing the diet long-term, or only until you meet your goals?
- How will you track the intake of macronutrients?
- What are your diet preferences?

Calculate Body Mass Index

Body Mass Index or BMI is an indicator of whether or not your current weight is healthy compared to your height. You can calculate your BMI by dividing your weight in kilograms by your squared height (m). If your results are between 18.5 and 24.9, you are healthy. Anything below 18.5 isn't healthy. The ideal measure is 21 for women and 23 for men. However, this calculation doesn't account for the body fat, waist circumference, your habits of eating, and your lifestyle. All of this goes into how healthy you are.

Your BMI can be higher if you are masculine, which doesn't mean that you should lose weight if you are healthy. You can think of yourself as obese if your BMI is over 30. However, this isn't exclusive to the number because it's possible to have a healthy weight with an unhealthy amount of body fat. These are rough calculations that can cause you to think of someone who is Athletic, as well as someone who is thinner but has more body fat as obese. However, calculating your BMI can help you determine your goals for weight loss in collaboration with your doctor and a dietitian.

Calculate the Body Fat Percentage

Looking into your body-fat percentage will help you to understand what you should do to lose weight, for example:

- Which method of Intermittent Fasting is the most appropriate?
- Whether or not you want to incorporate the Keto diet in the Intermittent Fasting?
- How much do you need to exercise, and what kind of exercises are necessary?

If you like exercising, Intermittent Fasting will help you lose body fat, but preserve or gain muscle mass. As a result, you may not notice scaling down. However, even if you don't lose weight, but gain muscle mass, you will still look slimmer.

To track how your body fat changes, you can use the body composition scales. These scales help you track how your muscle mass, your hydration, and your body fat change throughout your diet.

Calculate Waist-To-Hip Ratio

The waist-hip ratio or WHR is a more credible measurement because it accounts for your natural body shape. For women, an ideal measure is 0.8, while 0.9 is ideal for men. If your measurements are higher, you should work on your shape.

For calculating the WHR, you can use a tape measure and measure the circumference of the widest part of your hips and your natural waist, which is slightly above your belly button. After that, divide your waist measurement by your hip measurement.

Plan Your Portions

Calculate Basal Metabolic Rate

While measuring meals isn't required with Intermittent Fasting, it is desirable to maintain optimal health levels. To start, you should calculate your basal metabolic rate to find out how many calories you need to maintain your weight, and how many you need to lose it.

Calculate the Right Portion Sizes

When calculating portion sizes, keep in mind that 1 gram of nutrients translates to a different amount of calories:

- Fat-9 calories,
- Protein- 4 calories, and
- Carbohydrate-4 calories.

Calculate the Daily Calorie Intake

In general, Intermittent Fasting doesn't require calorie restriction for weight loss. Still, weight loss and other health benefits of fasting will be greater if you have a controlled daily calorie intake.

What to Expect

For most people who are starting with Intermittent Fasting, skipping breakfast is one of the most drastic changes. No matter how strange it might feel not to have breakfast, resist the temptation if the meal doesn't fit into your feeding window. Your appetite will be suppressed in the morning, and there's no use of eating if you're not hungry.

While most people don't experience severe hunger while fasting, it is possible to get occasional cravings. This happens because the majority of our eating is habitual. As a result of habitual eating, the balance of the hormones in charge of hunger and satiety is disturbed. The longer you fast, the better will these hormones balance out. As you regain a healthy sense of your body's natural appetite, habitual cravings will decrease.

It's also not recommended to eat late in the evening, despite intense cravings you might feel. Doing so will produce greater amounts of insulin because insulin is maximally stimulated with eating at this time. If you make dinner your largest meal, you will slow down the weight loss. Your largest meal should be around 3 p.m., while the evening meal should be lighter.

What to Look For

You can choose between numerous Intermittent Fasting variations. Some of the ways to determine the right fasting plan are to consider the following:

- Do you need to eat in the morning, or you can delay your first meal?
- Do you get hungry in the evening?
- Do you feel like you want to fast on certain days, but not the others?

Answering these questions will help you determine whether you want to fast daily, or you want to fast a certain number of days during a week and eat as usual during the remainder of the week.

Chapter 7: What to Eat During Intermittent Fasting?

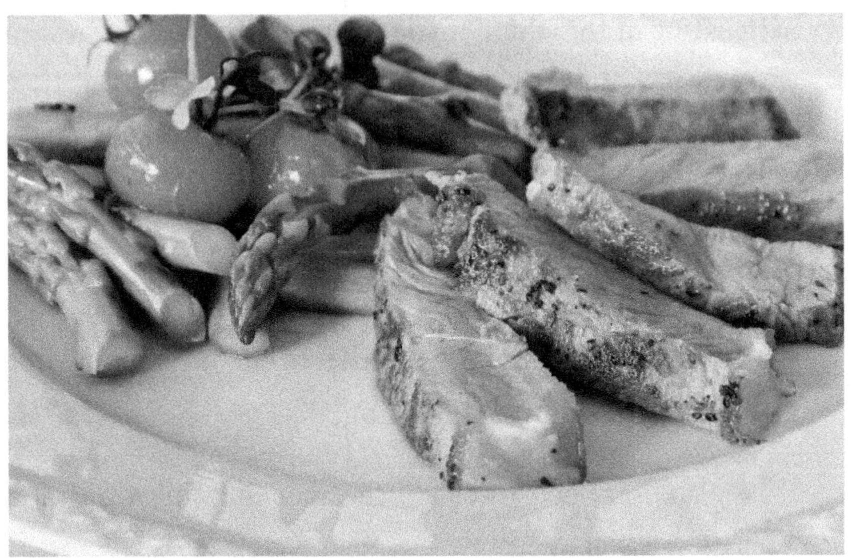

Now that you know why and how to practice Intermittent Fasting, it is time for you to learn how and what you should eat to regain your health. In this chapter, you will learn more about proper eating for Intermittent Fasting.

Recommendations and Nutrition Tips

The same health risks from an unhealthy diet are present with Intermittent Fasting. This means that to improve health with Intermittent Fasting, you'll also have to change the way you eat. The most prevalent illnesses of the modern world are diet-related. To start with your diet the right way, you want to establish a healthy eating patterns (Hamilton, 2017).

Control Fat Intake

General recommendations are for the fat to take up to 30% of your calorie intake. If you're going on a Keto diet, this percentage will be higher. The count of calories you consume isn't as relevant for weight loss as the composition of your meal. A better way to think about your diet is which specific foods you want to eat versus calories. If you're suffering from metabolic syndrome, it is essential to think about how certain foods will affect your glucose levels.

Remove sugars and reduce refined foods

It won't be completely possible to remove all sugars and processed foods from your diet. However, it is important for you to exclude snacks, sodas, cakes, pastries, and bottled/canned goods from your diet.

What to Eat

Eat whole foods

It is important to avoid processed foods if you want to reduce glucose successfully. When foods are being processed, they are deprived of the most nutritious parts and left only with carbohydrates. Processing completely disrupts the balance of micro and macronutrients, as well as fiber in foods. When foods are ground, that only speeds up the absorption of carbs into your bloodstream. The best foods are those in their natural state.

Eat Natural Fats

Healthy fats include salmon, avocados, olive oil, nuts, unprocessed meat, and dairy. These foods reduce the risks of heart disease and cardiometabolic disorders. But the type of fats to avoid are artificial fats. Healthy fats are healthy because they're raw, natural, and unprocessed. Their chemical composition hasn't been changed. Vegetable oils and baked goods are an example of bad fats because their composition has been altered by processing.

When foods are processed, they're exposed to chemicals to prolong the shelf life, and often other ingredients are added to enhance the flavor and color. It's no secret that many manufacturers will add vast amounts of cornstarch into the mix to achieve greater amounts of the product by using lesser amounts of primary ingredients. For example, if you take a look at the label of any bottle of a store-bought sauce, you'll notice that corn starch, food colors, and aromas, take up the major percentage of the content inside the bottle, while sourced ingredients (e.g., pesto, curry, tomato, or soy) often take up less than 20% of the mix. The biggest problem with artificial fats is that most of them are made from starchy ingredients, which all break down into glucose when digested.

If you purchase a bottle of the pesto sauce, which is healthy when homemade, you'll mainly eat liquid cornstarch with aromas, and barely 20-30% of the actual sauce. However, if you get virgin olive oil and organic cheeses for the sauce, you can make a healthy sauce that will contain healthy fats and won't increase risks from metabolic and heart disease.

What About the Cost?

Organic, healthy groceries seem to cost more, which is why many people believe they're a privilege of the rich. Keep in mind that, while the same amount of clean vs. processed groceries does cost more, it will be more satiating, and you'll most likely need smaller amounts to feel full and satisfied. The bigger issue is finding clean food since very few stores sell them at a fair price. If clean foods do seem out of your reach financially, you can think about gardening or ordering larger amounts of groceries from the nearest farm. It seems like a lot of effort with little to gain, but investing in healthy foods will reduce the costs of medication for treating symptoms of chronic illnesses, not to mention long-term improvements in mood and energy you're unlikely to achieve with medication and supplements.

What to Drink

Hydration remains equally important during your diet as it is in any other occasion. If you're recovering from chronic illness or working out intensely, hydration becomes even more important. The following sections will give you a more detailed explanation of what you should and shouldn't drink while you're fasting:

What to Drink While You're in a Fasted State
While you're in a fasted state, you should take abundant amounts of clean, mineral water, and so-called "non-caloric" drinks. These drinks include the following unsweetened and unprocessed tea and coffee.

What to Drink During Your Feeding Window
There's a bit more variety of drinks to consume while you're in a fed state. While this section won't cover all possible available beverages, you can make your own judgment calls, given that your drinks qualify as natural, healthy, unsweetened, and unprocessed. I suggest the following drinks:

- Coconut milk and water,
- Aloe-Vera-based beverages,
- Stevia,
- Apple-Cider vinegar,
- Tea and coffee,

- And others.

These beverages contain very little sugar, but are rich in vitamins and minerals that will have a replenishing effect on your body.

What to Drink During Non-Fasting Days

In general, no restrictions regarding beverages apply during non-fasting days. However, I would advise sticking to healthy options and avoiding excessive amounts of alcohol and sugary drinks. If you wish to treat yourself on non-fasting days, I'd suggest freshly squeezed fruit juices and smoothies. Still, keep in mind that fruit beverages can contain substantial amounts of sugar. Limit your fruit intake within the frames of healthy and reasonable.

Which Drinks You Should Avoid

Whether or not you're fasting, it would be wise to limit alcohol intake. In a fasted state, even a single alcoholic beverage might have a severe impact. Other than that, I suggest avoiding citrus juices, such as lemon and lime, during your fasting days. With a restricted calorie intake, the acidity of these drinks might cause stomach aches. Also, avoid sugary drinks like smoothies and sodas. These drinks will elevate your blood glucose and reduce the benefits of fasting.

Chapter 8: Intermittent Fasting and Diabetes

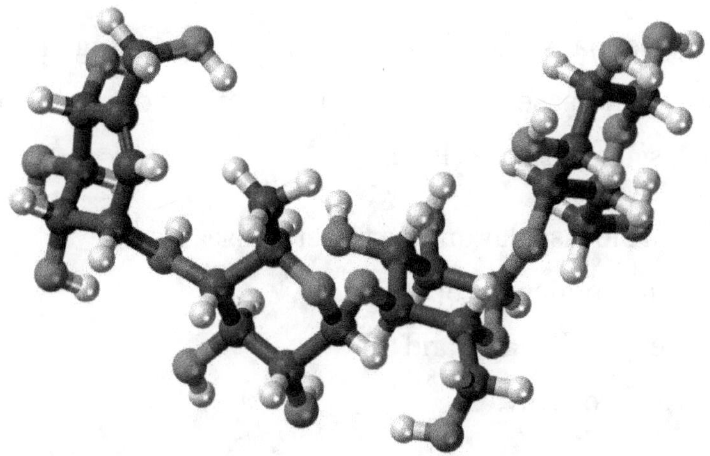

The rates of cardiometabolic disorders such as diabetes are steadily increasing, despite the medical advancements in treatments. In this chapter, you will learn more about diabetes and the effects of fasting on treating the disorder (Pace, 2017).

What is Diabetes Mellitus?

Diabetes Mellitus includes multiple metabolic disorders that involve either:

- Deficiency of insulin
- Decreased sensitivity to insulin

When there's insufficient insulin in the blood, the glucose doesn't move to the cells to supply them with energy. Instead, it remains in the blood. As a result, blood glucose rises above normal.

Hyperglycemia is a condition in which there are high levels of glucose. It increases the risk of complications of micro and macrovascular diseases like:

- Cardiovascular and peripheral diseases,
- Autonomic neuropathies,
- Retinal damage, and
- Nephropathy.

Type 2 diabetes is the most common form of Diabetes Mellitus, and mainly includes insulin resistance with some degree of insulin deficiency. Studies have shown that Intermittent Fasting can contribute to the weight loss that is similar to the result of the standard dietary changes recommended for people with Type 2 Diabetes. The majority of studies found a significant reduction in HbA1c (blood glucose level) with Intermittent Fasting compared to regular calorie restriction diets. One of the goals for healthcare professionals who treat those with diabetes is to modify the insulin on the pre-fasting and fasting days. This helps avoid hypoglycemia and manage the fasting regime safely.

Who is at risk of Type 2 Diabetes?

Typically, those who are obese and physically inactive throughout an extended period may develop diabetes, including people with a family history of Type 2 Diabetes. If type 2 diabetes is present in your family line, it is a cause for caution. However, even if there's no history of diabetes in your family, it is still possible to develop the disorder as a result of unhealthy eating habits or due to untreated hormonal disorders.

Type 2 diabetes is best treated by:

- Normalizing blood glucose levels and
- Minimizing low blood glucose levels for hypoglycemia and hyperglycemia.

Achieving the right blood glucose goals is the focus of the treatment, as well as:

- Diet and lifestyle counseling
- Medication
- Self-monitoring of blood glucose levels.
- Obesity is greatly associated with diabetes and the development of complications. In obese people, goals for the treatment of Type 2 diabetes include:
- Weight reduction (diet and lifestyle)
- Medication and surgery, and
- Treating microvascular and cardiovascular disease.

Diabetes and Diet

There's no single diet recommended to treat type 2 diabetes; the right diet depends on each individual, their preferences, and lifestyle. The best wait to tailor a diet for the treatment of diabetes is for a person to consult their healthcare team and consider all factors relevant to the diet. Your healthcare team should be familiar with a variety of diet plans and strategies for weight loss, the reduction of cardiovascular disease risks, and glycemic risks. General recommendations for dietary changes include:

- A reduction in energy intake
- Modifying eating behaviors
- Modifying eating patterns.

The following diets have proven effective in helping people who suffer from Type 2 Diabetes:

- Low carbohydrate,
- High protein,
- Very low calorie, and
- Low glycemic index diets.

Recommended diet changes for diabetes include a nutrient-dense, healthy eating plan to normalize blood glucose, blood pressure, and lipid profile.

Dietary changes can greatly improve the health of those with type 2 diabetes. When creating a diet plan, it is important for both you and your healthcare team to design a sustainable, realistic plan that will account for your habits, preferences, work, and lifestyle. It is important to consider:

- Individual needs and preferences,
- Culture, and
- Knowledge and understanding of medical and nutritional terms.

Practical and supportive self-management in battling type 2 diabetes is important for long-term progress.

Diabetes and Fasting

Intermittent Fasting is often recommended for those who have type 2 diabetes. The terms "Intermittent Fasting" and "alternate-day fasting" refer to the number of days per week during which the person will be fasting. Intermittent Fasting for diabetes usually includes a 70-75% calorie reduction on fasting days, which is similar to following a healthy weight loss plan of 500-600kcal with an approximately 25% of calorie restriction.

Numerous types of Intermittent Fasting, such as intermittent energy restriction and time-restricted feeding, have become a topic of interest when it comes to treating diabetes. They are based on the assumption that to lose weight, a person doesn't need to restrict calories every day.

Insulin resistance has been considered to be a common factor in underlying risks from cardio-metabolic diseases. Insulin resistance is a state in which the body produces less insulin to create a biological effect, which results in interruptions in glucose homeostasis that can cause type 2 diabetes. Insulin resistance can happen in different tissues, including skeletal tissues, muscle, liver and adipose tissues. Deposition of ectopic fat may arise from increased eating, and impaired adipose tissue storage also contribute to developing insulin resistance.

Ingesting the food and the influx of nutrients that follows, mainly glucose and arginine into the bloodstream, stimulates the secretion of insulin from pancreatic beta cells. This mechanism is one of the most important mechanisms for the regulation of glucose after eating.

Peripheral insulin resistance is one of the most signs of type two diabetes. It has four stages:

- Compensatory hyperinsulinemia after eating,
- Hyperinsulinemia and hyperglycemia after eating,
- Elevated insulin during fasting and high glucose levels, and
- Development of type two diabetes.

Common dietary changes to treat type 2 diabetes include:

- Fasting for 1-3 days/week,
- Reducing the energy intake to 60-80% on fasting days, and
- Eating one meal or several smaller meals during the fasting days.

No calorie restriction is required on the non-fasting days. Still, the general recommendations for healthy eating apply, especially when it comes to controlling sugar intake to normalize blood sugar levels.

Hypoglycemia is a risk for those with type 2 diabetes for those who are on a low-carbohydrate diet, which is why it is critically important for anyone with diabetes not to reduce their food intake without consulting their doctor. When the calorie intake isn't planned and advised by an expert, it's usually ineffective.

When it comes to obesity, the rates have more than doubled during the recent decades. Obesity is associated with numerous metabolic complications, which increase the risk of cardiometabolic diseases, such as type two diabetes and cardiovascular disease. The rates of these diseases are increasing. Weight management and calorie restriction have been considered significant factors to reduce risks.

Chapter 9: Intermittent Fasting and Women

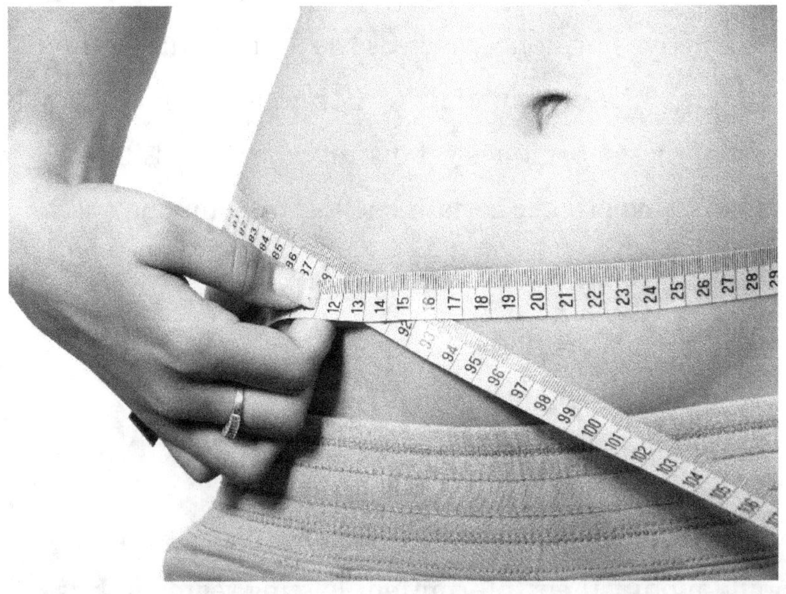

While the evidence of the health benefits of Intermittent Fasting applies equally to men and women, there is some evidence that women respond to fasting differently. Some studies show that blood glucose levels may worsen in women who have fasted for over three weeks, and there is also evidence that Intermittent Fasting may disturb the menstrual cycle. However, these findings were limited to those women who are more sensitive to calorie restriction than the majority (Hamilton, 2017).

Calorie restriction isn't required in Intermittent Fasting but may happen accidentally if the diet isn't properly managed and monitored. As a result of calorie restriction, the hypothalamus, a part of the brain, may reduce the secretion of the hormone GnRH, which is in charge of releasing Gonadotropin. This hormone impacts the release of female reproductive hormones, such as the follicle-stimulating hormone (FSH) and luteinizing hormone (LH). When normal levels of these hormones get disrupted, it is possible for women to experience certain health problems such as:

- Infertility,
- Irregular periods,
- Impaired bone health,
- And others.

To avoid hormonal imbalances and health risks, women should modify their Intermittent Fasting regimen. It is recommended for women to choose fewer fasting days and shorter periods of fasting, which means that the best Intermittent Fasting options for women are:

- 12-hour fast,
- 16-hour fast,
- Eat-stop-eat,
- The 5:2 fast, and
- The Leangains Method.

Numerous studies have also shown that women tend to experience the side-effects of Intermittent Fasting more intensely than men. Women are more prone to headaches, mood swings, hunger, bad breath, and a decline in concentration.

In general, fasting is not recommended or recommended only with medical guidance, to women who have a history of diabetes, eating disorders, low sugar levels, nutrient deficiency, or are underweight. Women who are trying to get pregnant, are pregnant or are breastfeeding shouldn't fast.

Chapter 10: Intermittent Fasting and Training

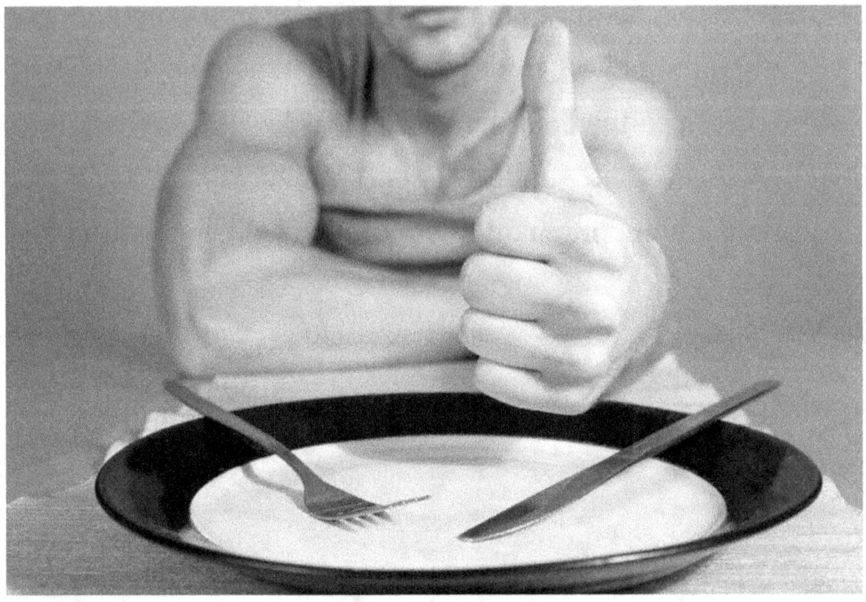

Exercise has been proven to boost the effects of Intermittent Fasting (Moore & Fung, 2017). The research has shown that exercise, while not essential for weight loss with Intermittent Fasting, can:

- Intensify the fat burning;
- Stimulate the growth of muscle cells and tissues;
- Help the body detoxify;

What does the research say about exercise during Intermittent Fasting?

- **Improved body composition and insulin resistance**

Effects of exercise during Intermittent Fasting showed that a 15-week high-intensity exercise regimen had an impact on trunk fat and insulin resistance. Those who exercised intensely while fasting has shown a significant reduction in fat storages, but also an improvement (a reduction of) insulin resistance greater than those who've fasted without exercise. High-intensity exercise at a medically safe and expertly managed pace can help you reduce total body fat, leg, and trunk fat, as well as reduce insulin resistance.

- **Improved athletic performance**

Another study showed that fasting during the month of Ramadan could have both positive and negative impacts on athletic performance. Ramadan fasting didn't seem to affect physical performance and weight and didn't have any exercise effect on the exercise, and there wasn't a decrease in physical performance. All athletes who were studied had regular physical activity, which includes moderate exercise.

Some negative impact was recorded amongst runners, mainly affecting speed and agility and enduring endurance in soccer players. However, these results can be attributed to other factors outside the diet, such as the physical condition and the habits of training.

- **Better muscle growth**

One study showed that the participants grew more muscle when they trained while they were in a fasted state. Intermittent Fasting is often used by weight-training enthusiasts as a technique to boost muscles and burn fat. The research has shown that aerobic training during the fasted state will help you burn more fat. Some studies also suggest that exercising while fasting will help burn body fat and build your muscles. However, a diet rich in protein is important because your muscles grow out of your protein intake.

When to Train While Fasting

Integrating exercise into Intermittent Fasting often seems confusing. As you've learned by now, there's no reason to fear that exercising while fasting will have negative consequences to your health, or cause additional strain to your body. However, there are a couple of smart tips to follow if you want to speed up weight loss and improve your shape while fasting. If you're unsure how to schedule your meal around exercise, start by adjusting your feeding window to the training intensity. Here are a couple of ways to do it:

Light Cardio Exercise

If you prefer short cardio exercises, like a 30-minute running session, you can do this in a fasted state. This means that you have to eat neither before nor after training. However, if training, while you're in a fasted state, causes you to feel weak or dizzy, don't hesitate to have a snack.

Intense Cardio Exercise

More intense exercise routines are best done while you're in a fed state. Intense training will take some supply of stored glycogen to support intense training. In this case, make sure to adjust your calorie intake to support extra activity and exercise on a full stomach.

If you're a training enthusiast or a professional, it is best to exercise in a fed state. However, this doesn't mean that you should overeat before training. Instead, you should have a small meal or a snack 2-3 hours before exercising, and no later than 20 minutes before. You can make your pre-training meal rich in carbohydrates, but you don't have to if you're following the Ketogenic diet.

How to Train While Fasting

Schedule Training Around Your Diet

It is essential to schedule your exercises around the feeding times so that you have one meal up to three hours before and after exercising. The intense exercise followed by fasting may result in the loss of muscle tissue.

Increase Protein and Carbohydrates

The more intense your exercise, the more protein you'll need. Sufficient protein will help you build healthy, strong muscles, and it won't slow down the process of burning fat. If you prefer intense strength training, make sure to have a meal containing carbohydrates and at least 20 grams of protein after exercise, preferably within an hour.

Drink Water and Supply Electrolytes

Hydration is important when fasting, and even more important while training. To compensate for the loss of water and electrolytes after exercise, make sure to have enough water or coconut water.

Adjust Exercise to the Fasting Type

The rule of thumb is that your exercise should reduce in intensity as your fasting time increases. This means that you should practice more intensely if your fasting times are shorter, and practice low-intensity activities like walking or yoga if your fast lasts longer than 24 hours.

Follow Your Instincts

Your safety and well-being come first. If, at any time during exercise, you start to feel weak or hungry, lower the intensity of the training, and have a small meal. Following the cues of your body will help you avoid accidents, preserve muscle tissue, and prevent any harm to come from an extreme calorie deficit.

Chapter 11: Intermittent Fasting and the Keto Diet

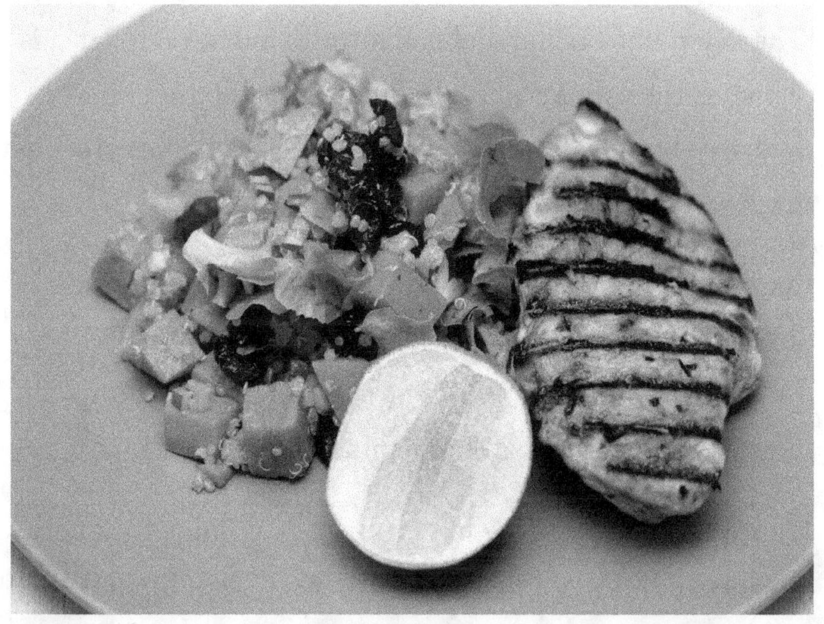

The Ketogenic diet was designed in the 1930s at the May Clinic in Rochester, Minnesota. It was designed for children who have epilepsy and has proven effective in reducing and preventing seizures. Quickly after its creation, the diet became popular in treating adults. Nowadays, the ketogenic diet is no longer used only for medical purposes. With scientifically recorded benefits of restricting carbohydrates and protein, and increasing the intake of fat up to 90%, the diet is now widely used, researched, and debated (Perillo, 2019). Combined with Intermittent Fasting, this diet was proven to support weight loss and contribute to less acidosis and hypoglycemia. It's been noted that the flexibility in the diet regarding calorie intake didn't reduce its benefits.

How Does the Keto Diet Work?

The ketogenic fasting diet is known to induce ketogenesis, which is the process of producing ketone bodies, beta-hydroxy-butyrate, and acetoacetate. These bodies are created from fatty acids in the liver.

As well as directly affecting the creation and the release of ketone bodies, the diet was also shown to impact the nutrient-integrating pathways. Meaning, the diet impacts how the body processes nutrients and burns fat.

There are two ways in which your body obtains the energy it needs to supply your cells and organs. One of them is by using the carbohydrates, and the other one is by using fats. When your body uses fats instead of carbohydrates, it used the bodies called ketones that are created in the liver. Ketones release when your body metabolizes food and breaks down fatty acids.

Metabolism refers to chemical reactions inside the body that work even when you're sleeping. One way for your body to fuel metabolism is by the use of glucose that is created once your body breaks down carbohydrates from food. The problem with glucose is that your body will crave more food once these supplies in the blood run out.

Changing your diet to a low-carbohydrate, high-fat, and high-protein will allow your body to get into a state of ketosis. When you're in ketosis, your body will metabolize fat and trigger the release of ketones. To achieve this, it is recommended that fats make between 60 and 80 percent of the daily calorie intake, between 20 and 30 percent of protein, and 5 to 10 percent of carbs.

Net carbohydrates

Carbohydrates are present in all foods to some degree, which makes it impossible to exclude them from your diet completely. To stay healthy, you shouldn't eliminate fiber from your diet. You will get the net carbohydrate measure when you subtract the total fiber calorie count from the total number of carbs the food contains. However, for the diet to be successful, you need to account for the fiber as your carbohydrate intake.

Ketogenic diet and Intermittent Fasting

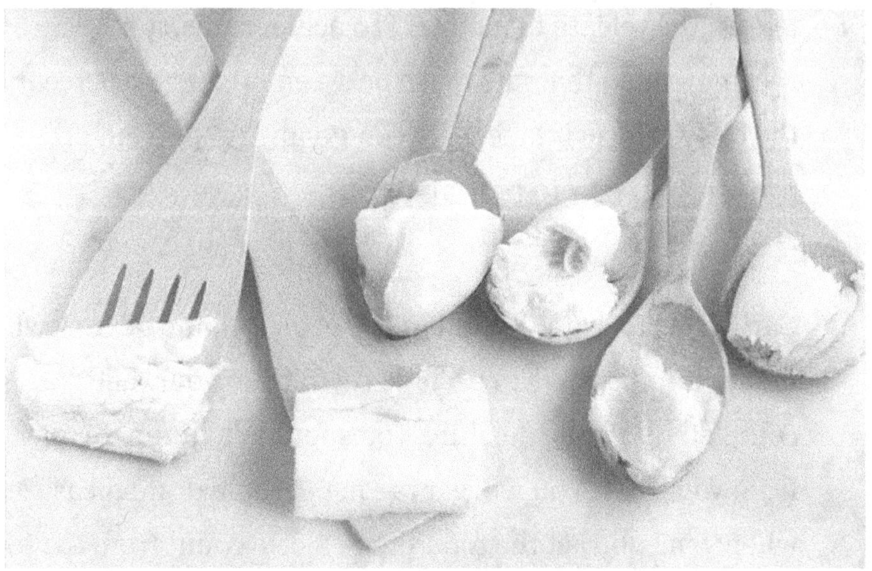

When the ketogenic diet is combined with Intermittent Fasting, the meals are consumed during a feeding window. Normally, the ketogenic diet doesn't entail any particular timings of meals or spacing out meals to a certain amount of time. However, when fasting on the keto diet, you will alter the composition of your meals to increase the intake of fat and proteins and reduce carbohydrates.

It will take some time for the process of ketosis to start, usually between one and three days. In some people, the process might take up to a week. Your activity levels, diet, and weight will affect the speed of entering ketosis. To achieve the state of ketosis, your body will first have to use up all of its glucose supplies. Once these supplies run out, your body will automatically switch to burning fat. When this happens, your liver will start releasing ketones. In the initial stage of ketosis, your ketone levels will be low. You might begin to feel the symptoms of the keto flu. The longer you stay in the state of ketosis, the easier the symptoms will be.

It is possible to feel certain cravings during the initial stages of the diet. Naturally, you might get hungry during these times of the day when you'd usually eat, like early morning or late evening. However, these cravings should reduce with enough persistence. When you're combining Intermittent Fasting with the ketogenic diet, your body continuously creates ketones by burning fat, but with a prolonged amount of time to put this process into action. This way, you are maximizing the processes of burning fat and healing your body, and your body is burning fat more efficiently without losing muscle mass.

Still, switching from regular to the ketogenic diet is a major change. For this reason, it is recommended to start with the ketogenic diet first, and then move onto fasting. This way, your body will have enough time to adjust, and the change won't be as drastic.

First, make sure to be considerate of your eating times. Start by gradually establishing a feeding window that is most appropriate. To check the number of ketones, you can choose between doing a blood test, urine test, or a breath test. The blood test is the most reliable method, but it is also the most expensive.

When incorporating the ketogenic diet into Intermittent Fasting, you should have around 160g of fat, 70g of protein, and 20g of carbohydrates on an average 1800-calorie diet. When you're dieting for weight loss (1500 calories), you should have 130g of fat, 60g of protein, and 20g of carbohydrates.

The most challenging part of the keto diet is to replace the foods that are common and most satisfying. Here are a couple of suggested alternatives:

- Pasta: Shirataki noodles, zoodles, spaghetti squash
- Flower: pork cracklings, unprocessed and unsweetened coconut flakes, almond flour.
- Rice: Shirataki and Cauliflower ice.
- Milk: Cheese and heavy cream.
- Bread: Keto bread, low-carb tortillas.
- Fries and sweet potato: Zucchini fries.
- Citruses and fruits: Lemon and limes
- Beans: Eggs, seafood, poultry and meat.
- Sweeteners: monk fruit, stevia.
- Oil: olive, coconut, avocado, sesame, butter, ghee.

On the other hand, you want to avoid sugary drinks, root vegetables, processed foods, and refined sugars. An easy way to decide if you should have a particular vegetable is to think about whether it grows above or beneath the ground.

If you're just starting with the keto diet, here are some suggestions for your first shopping list:

- Meat: bacon, sausage, eggs, heavy cream, butter, beef, pork, fish, poultry;
- Nuts and seeds: coconut, almonds, walnuts, pecans, brazil nuts, chia seeds, etc.
- Canned and fermented foods: coconut and almond cream and milk, olives, unprocessed dark chocolate, stevia, tea, coffee, full-fat plain yogurt, sauerkraut, kimchi, and pickles.
- Sweeteners and spices: red pepper, oregano, basil, smoked paprika, bay leaves, black pepper, sea salt, curry powder, mustard (whole grain), monk fruit sweetener (unsweetened).

While the highest amount of protein in the ketogenic diet commonly comes from meat, eggs, fish, and dairy are a good alternative for those who are vegetarian. Gathering recipes is a good way to start the diet because it will help you customize your meal plan.

The Risks of the Ketogenic Diet

The Ketogenic diet can have adverse health effects, mainly because it restricts the intake of many nutrient-dense vegetables (e.g., carrots, potatoes, dairy, root vegetables, and fruit). It also carries a risk of vitamin and mineral deficiency, as well as hypercholesterolemia, acidosis, and constipation.

To protect against these risks, it is important to avoid calorie restriction and take proper supplementation. It is recommended to take Vitamin D, calcium, selenium, and zinc.

Aside from epilepsy, the ketogenic diet was found to be effective in battling Alzheimer's, migraines, Parkinson's, brain injuries, and autism. Many studies have shown that the ketogenic diet contributed to the improvement of the symptoms.

The ketogenic diet is often used in combination with Intermittent Fasting. The diet itself is made to create similar effects of fasting and have the best effects when combined with Intermittent Fasting.

Chapter 12: Tips for Successful Intermittent Fasting

As you reach the end of this book, you know how to practice Intermittent Fasting, and you've probably become aware of the method that suits you best. In this chapter, I will give you a couple of additional tips for successful Intermittent Fasting.

1. Maintain the right mindset

Fasting is all about allowing your body to tell you when you're physically hungry. Fad diets don't allow that because you are eating habitually when your body doesn't need food. You are also working against metabolic mechanisms that want you to store fat to supply energy for times of starvation.

2. Be mindful about your hunger

In one of the previous sections of this book, you learned about possible causes of your appetite that aren't related to true physical hunger. If appetite and cravings pose a true challenge, keep a food journal and track your appetite. Not the times of the day when you feel hungriest, and think about the possibility that your cravings might be habitual or emotional. If you are otherwise healthy, I would recommend trying to tolerate the appetite as long as you don't feel (Perillo, 2019):

- Weakness, dizziness, and fatigue;
- Shivering, sweating, or cold; or
- Any other type of distress.

3. Never ignore warning signs

If you are considering going on a fasting regimen, and you are treating for any form of diabetes, cardiometabolic illness or any other chronic illness, put your safety first. No matter how bad it feels to break your fast, never ignore your hunger. Your health comes first, and I advise against tolerating hunger if you suspect that your health might suffer.

4. Communicate with your healthcare team

Run all of your ideas, questions, suggestions, or concerns by your doctor and dietitian. While this book provided sufficient information for you to understand how fasting works and how to apply it, your healthcare team knows you best. They are familiar with your specific health conditions, dietary needs, lifestyle, preferences, and desirable changes. While I did my best to present you with useful ways to plan your diet and meals, and most practical methods for you fast, your healthcare team will suggest the simplest and most sustainable meal options. They'll make it easier for you to understand how much, what, and when to eat for effective Intermittent Fasting.

5. Stay hydrated

Non-caloric beverages, such as unsweetened, unprocessed tea, coffee, and water will help you feel fresh and stay energized during the fasting period. Don't ignore your body's need for liquids. Doing so could lead to dehydration, weakness, dizziness, and fatigue.

6. Start slow and stay private

While Intermittent Fasting can be considered a well-researched diet, it is still misunderstood by many. I suggest taking advice only from qualified experts, and not allowing criticism and doubts from those who don't understand fasting to get to you. If your health situation is complicated, your friends and family might fear that you're taking unnecessary risks by fasting. However, if your doctor thinks that this method is a good way for you to lose weight and improve well-being, save both yourself and loved ones from stress by keeping your diet private.

If you like feeling connected and supported, you can always reach out to online or local communities and support groups that practice fasting. That said, give yourself enough time to learn and adapt to the new diet. I advise against starting with long fasts that last more than six hours. Instead, start by fasting 2-3 days of the week, preferably on the days when you're not very active. Once your body adapts to the fast, you can move on to longer or regular fasting.

Chapter 13: Frequently Asked Questions

In this chapter, I will answer some of the most frequent questions about Intermittent Fasting (Moore & Fung, 2017). These answers will help you relieve some of the doubts about the right ways to eat, manage your hunger, and exercise during your diet.

When Should I Eat?

The majority of studies suggest eating earlier during the day. This is because your body becomes more insulin resistant in the evening. That said, there are multiple methods of Intermittent Fasting that set the feeding window during the evening hours. If you have trouble with late-night hunger, you can consider 24-hour fasting or the Warrior diet. However, if these fasts are too intense for you, you can always choose the 5:2 or 4:3 fasting, which will allow you to eat during the day. In this case, I suggest making your mid-day meal the largest, and having a smaller meal or a snack in the evening.

What Should I Eat on Non-Fasting Days?

I suggest maintaining a healthy, nutrient-dense diet even when you're not fasting. The only differences between your fasting and non-fasting days are in the timing and the size of your meals. On fasting days, you'll eat one large or multiple smaller meals. However, when you're not fasting, I still suggest avoiding sugar and processed foods.

Will Exercising Be Hard With Fasting?

Most people are concerned about exercising when fasting. I will remind you that the majority of reliable studies showed that fasting wouldn't impair your physical ability to exercise, nor will exercise make it harder to fast. However, I suggest adjusting the size of your meals to eat more on your workout days. You want to avoid calorie deprivation and the loss of muscle mass, which can happen if you eat the same amount of food as usual, but burn more calories due to exercise.

How Long Should I Fast?

You can fast until you reach your health and weight loss goals and then stop. There would be no adverse effects on your health and weight if your diet during the fast were adequate. If you remember the study of the impact of Ramadan fast on weight loss from Chapter 1, you'll remember that the study participants regained their weight after the fast. This happened because their diet was inadequate. It was rich in carbohydrates and lacked protein. As a result, the participants mainly lost water weight and muscle mass. If you don't want this to happen, be mindful of your diet and prioritize protein, fats, fiber, and an abundance of vegetables over carbs. This will ensure long-term weight loss. Other than that, quitting Intermittent Fasting won't have negative consequences on your weight and health if you address and change your negative eating habits. If you stop eating out of stress and boredom and learn to resist unhealthy foods, quitting the fast shouldn't have negative outcomes.

How to Cope With Hunger?

You shouldn't feel hungry while fasting if you've taken sufficient calories during your feeding time. That said, it is usual for people to feel hungry up to 10 days after they've begun fasting. This happens because Ghrelin, your hunger hormone, isn't impacted by fasting. Instead, time-limited eating affects Leptin, a hormone that makes you feel full. Your hunger will trigger habitually, or due to hormonal imbalance. Once the two hormones start regaining balance, you will only feel hungry when your body needs food. You should always prioritize well-being over a diet regimen. But, if you feel like tolerating a certain degree of hunger won't put you at risk, you can always have a cup of coffee or tea to relieve the cravings.

Conclusion

In this book, I tried to present you with a simple but studious explanation of Intermittent Fasting and its benefits to the human body. I want to thank you for staying with me throughout the entire book. Hopefully, you've learned enough about Intermittent Fasting and its healing potential to start practicing the diet, and unlock the healing mechanisms within your body. Throughout this book, my goal was to inform about the real, science-based facts and findings to alleviate some of the fears and concerns surrounding Intermittent Fasting. The explanations and instructions in this book have, hopefully, showed you that fasting is simple, easy and safe.

In this book, you also learned that by fasting you could trigger self-healing processes inside your own body and start healing and rejuvenating. With the simple act of framing your daily meals into a limited amount of time, you can unlock your body's hidden potential to shed old, unnecessary, and malfunctioning cells, and start to repair itself. Moreover, you now understand how Intermittent Fasting can help you lose weight rapidly and permanently. One of the goals of this book was to explain better how the conventional way of eating kept your fat storages locked away and to show you what you can do to start burning fat right now.

Last, but not least, this book presented you with the explanations for how Intermittent Fasting can help you recover from numerous chronic illnesses, such as heart disease, diabetes, insulin resistance and many more. As you start to make the positive changes suggested in this book, remember to stay mindful, patient, and careful with your own health and body. Remember to lean into your support system, and consult your physician before introducing any drastic changes into your diet.

Bibliography

Alayafi, Y. R. (2014). *The Physiological effect of intermittent fasting (fasting the month of Ramadan) on anthropometerics and blood varaibles* (Doctoral dissertation, University of Kansas).

Antoni, R. (2017). *Metabolic effects of intermittent fasting* (Doctoral dissertation, University of Surrey).

Berardi, J. M., Scott-Dixon, K., & Green, N. (2011). Experiments with Intermittent Fasting. *Toronto: Precision Nutrition.*

Hamilton, A. (2017). *Eat, Fast, Slim: The Life-Changing Intermittent Fasting Diet for Amazing Weight Loss and Optimum Health.* Watkins Media Limited.

Levine, B., & Klionsky, D. J. (2017). Autophagy wins the 2016 Nobel Prize in Physiology or Medicine: Breakthroughs in baker's yeast fuel advances in biomedical research. *Proceedings of the National Academy of Sciences, 114*(2), 201-205.

Mansell, K., Bowen, M., & Arnason, T. (2016). The Effects of Intermittent Fasting and a High-Protein Diet on Biochemical and Anthropometric Measurements in Type 2 Diabetes Mellitus. *Canadian Journal of Diabetes, 40*(5), S64.

Mosley, M., & Spencer, M. (2015). *The FastDiet-revised & updated: Lose weight, stay healthy, and live longer with the simple secret of intermittent fasting.* Simon and Schuster.

Moore, J., & Fung, J. (2016). *The complete guide to fasting: Heal your body through intermittent, alternate-day, and extended fasting.* Simon and Schuster.

Pace, K. A. (2017). *A feasibility study to investigate the effectiveness and safety of an intermittent fasting diet for weight reduction in adults with Type 2 Diabetes treated with insulin: a thesis presented in partial fulfilment of the requirements for the degree of Master of Science in Human Nutrition at Massey University, Albany, New Zealand* (Doctoral dissertation, Massey University).

Perillo, J. (2019). *The Beginner's Guide to Intermittent Keto: Combine the Powers of Intermittent Fasting with a Ketogenic Diet to Lose Weight and Feel Great*

Stephens, J. (2017). *Delay, Don't Deny: Living an Intermittent Fasting Lifestyle*